WHAT EVERY SPEECH–LANGUAGE PATHOLOGIST/AUDIOLOGIST SHOULD KNOW ABOUT SERVICE-LEARNING

Jennifer Kent-Walsh
University of Central Florida

Boston   Columbus   Indianapolis   New York   San Francisco   Upper Saddle River
Amsterdam   Cape Town   Dubai   London   Madrid   Milan   Munich   Paris   Montreal   Toronto
Mexico City   São Paulo   Sydney   Hong Kong   Seoul   Singapore   Taipei   Tokyo

Executive Editor and Publisher: Stephen D. Dragin
Editorial Assistant: Jamie Bushell
Marketing Manager: Weslie Sellinger
Production Editor: Karen Mason
Manufacturing Buyer: Megan Cochran
Cover Administrator: Diane Lorenzo

Library of Congress Cataloging-in-Publication Data

Kent-Walsh, Jennifer.
  What every speech–language pathologist/audiologist should know about service-learning / Jennifer Kent-Walsh.
    p. ; cm.
  Includes bibliographical references.
  ISBN-13: 978-0-13-248595-1
  ISBN-10: 0-13-248595-8
  I. Title.
  [DNLM: 1. Audiology--education. 2. Speech-Language Pathology--education. 3. Community-Institutional Relations. 4. Social Responsibility. WL 18]

  616.85'5--dc23

                                                    2011035182

1 2 3 V088 13 12 11

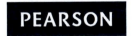

ISBN-10: 0-13-248595-8
ISBN-13: 978-0-13-248595-1

CONTENTS

ABOUT THE AUTHOR

Jennifer Kent-Walsh, Ph.D., CCC-SLP, S-LP(C), is an Associate Professor in the Department of Communication Sciences and Disorders at the University of Central Florida (UCF). In addition to conducting research and teaching undergraduate and graduate courses in augmentative and alternative communication (AAC) and language disorders, Dr. Kent-Walsh is the Director of the Florida Alliance for Assistive Services and Technology (FAAST) Atlantic Region Assistive Technology Demonstration Center at UCF. Dr. Kent-Walsh and her research collaborator, Cathy Binger, Ph.D., conduct research relating to the development and evaluation of interventions to improve language and communication outcomes for children with developmental disabilities who use AAC. Dr. Kent-Walsh also regularly teaches service-learning courses and conducts research to evaluate outcomes of service-learning in higher education.

ACKNOWLEDGMENTS

I would like to extend my sincere thanks to the many students who have shown great enthusiasm and engagement while completing service-learning projects over the years and to the many community partners with whom I have had the privilege to work. Special thanks to Carolyn Buchanan and Jessica Brown for their assistance with the preparation of this book. Finally, thanks to the faculty and staff of the Karen L. Smith Faculty Center for Teaching and Learning and the Office of Experiential Learning at the University of Central Florida for providing sustained support and resources for service-learning activities.

Jennifer Kent-Walsh

1

WHAT IS SERVICE-LEARNING?

When you chose to take a course or pursue a career in communication sciences and disorders (CSD), it is probable that the clinical aspects of our field played a large part in your decision-making process. Whether you were just interested in becoming more informed or you already knew you wanted to choose speech–language pathology or audiology as your professional field, you likely thought about the potential for working directly with individuals with communication disorders or the potential to help people indirectly.

Perhaps you had a personal experience with a specific type of client or communication disorder, such as a relative who had a stroke or a sibling with a hearing impairment, or perhaps you had an interest in working in a particular type of setting, like a hospital or school. Another possibility is that you had chosen to pursue a career in a related field like nursing or education and you decided to take a course in communication sciences and disorders to further your understanding of the types of patients, clients, or students with whom you will eventually work, or to further your knowledge of a group of professional colleagues with whom you will eventually collaborate. Regardless of the path that led you take a CSD course, it is likely that you have a desire to gain a depth of understanding and experience in the topic of the course.

We all know there is much that can be learned in classes, textbooks, modules, and laboratories. However, the experiences that students gain beyond these traditional educational media often are those they describe as involving "aha moments" or as "finally" bringing perspective to the content of the course. When students have hands-on experiences, they often talk about course content *coming alive* and seeming *real*. This brings us to the topic at hand in this book—service-learning. Service-learning is one mechanism that can help students to gain practical field-based experience within the context of any number of courses in speech–language pathology and audiology. Service-learning projects can involve a range of activities from more traditional or familiar clinical experiences to more unusual experiences that are not necessarily core requirements of an educational program in speech–language pathology or audiology from the perspective of our accrediting body, the American-Speech-Language-Hearing Association.

To help you gain a thorough understanding of service-learning, we will talk in this chapter about (a) definitions of service-learning and (b) key elements of service-learning.

Defining Service-Learning

Before considering the definition of service-learning per se, let's separately look at the two words "service" and "learning." The most relevant definitions you might identify via Dictionary.com (2011b) for "service" would likely be "an act of helpful activity" (noun) or "to supply with aid, information, or other incidental services" (verb). Similarly, either of the following definitions for "learning" may seem relevant to the concept of service-learning as well: (1) "knowledge acquired by systematic study in a field of scholarly application," or (2) "the act or process of acquiring knowledge or skill" (Dictionary.com, 2011a). After reassuring yourself that you are familiar with these two rather simple definitions, you may assume that you can infer an accurate definition of service-learning. Perhaps you have synergistic thoughts of students engaging in activities that allow them to gain knowledge or skills as they provide some type of assistance to another person or organization. Although there is widespread agreement on this type of basic underlying premise for service-learning, there is anything but widespread agreement on a complete definition for service-learning.

The variability in definitions for service-learning may be at least partially related to the fact that service-learning can take place at any level of education. Each school or institution that includes service-learning within the curriculum tends to adopt or develop a slightly different definition of the term. To put this in perspective, consider the following examples of academic service-learning projects and activities across the educational spectrum and see if you can identify some common components within each description.

- **Pre-kindergarten students,** learning about the life cycle and compassion in the community, plant vegetables in the school garden and after tending to the crops over time, donate the grown vegetables to a local soup kitchen.
- **Elementary school students,** learning about disease control and prevention, prepare colorful visual reminders of hygienic practices to be posted in their school and community center as reminders of how children can prevent the spread of illness.
- **Middle school students,** learning about anti-bullying and diversity, research and demonstrate social skills and techniques to end bullying and promote disability awareness using skits performed for younger students.
- **High school students,** learning about cancer in a biology course, organize a fundraiser to help support chemotherapy treatment for a local child and for a child in a developing country.
- **College students,** learning about human development in a psychology course, perform developmental screenings for children in a homeless shelter.
- **Undergraduate students,** learning about technical writing in a university English class, prepare policy and procedure manuals for nonprofit organizations.
- **Graduate students,** learning about interventions for individuals who are deaf and hard of hearing in a university speech–language pathology class, partner with a parent support group to prepare and offer family workshops on aural habilitation techniques.

You may have expected to see evidence of active learning in the above descriptions and you may not have been surprised by the obvious connections between the described activities and the identified course content or goals, but did you expect to note the common thread of activities that aimed to address specific community needs? These are the types of distinctions that are essential when attempting to differentiate service-learning from volunteerism or other forms of experiential learning with which you may be familiar.

The National Service-Learning Clearinghouse (2011b) delineates some of the aspects of service-learning that cut across educational contexts in the following definition:

> *Service-learning is a teaching and learning strategy that integrates meaningful community service with instruction and reflection to enrich the learning experience, teach civic responsibility, and strengthen communities.*

You can likely see how this definition could be applied to any of the above-described projects at various levels of education.

As an example of an institutionally adopted approach to service-learning in the specific context of higher education, consider the following definition, which is in place at the University of Central Florida (2011):

> *Service-learning is a teaching method that uses community involvement to apply theories or skills being taught in a course. Service-learning furthers the learning objectives of the academic course, addresses community needs, and requires students to reflect on their activity in order to gain an appreciation for the relationship between civics and academics.*

This definition of academic service-learning is contextualized within academic courses specifically and includes direct and implied emphasis on several elements that are commonly included in definitions of service-learning: (a) close connections with academic content via course objectives, (b) active reflection on the learning experience, (c) authentic community needs, and (d) meaningful service. Figure 1.1 illustrates the suggested cyclical relationship between each of these elements and how the elements converge within service-learning experiences. Although each element in the model can stand alone, it is the synergistic convergence of these elements that yields exciting service-learning opportunities. The University of Central Florida (2011) suggests that this convergence allows communities to receive an infusion of people power and access to university resources that then enables them to explore new ideas and generate energy in the context of civic responsibility. In addition to noting the convergence of these critical elements, it also is important to note that the interdependent relationship between service and learning is emphasized by the hyphen between the two words in the term itself. It has been suggested that the inclusion of the hyphen can be seen as symbolic of service-learning being realized via service and learning goals that are weighted equally and in a mutually enhancing manner (Eyler and Giles, 1999).

Figure 1.1

Model of Academic Service-Learning

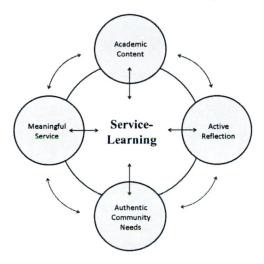

Essential Elements of Service-Learning

In order for service-learning experiences to be meaningful and successful, a number of essential elements have been proposed in the literature, including those inherent in the above model. A range of authors (e.g., Berger Kaye, 2004; Eyler & Giles, 1994, 1999; Mabry, 1998) have argued that careful consideration and planning related to essential service-learning elements can "make or break" student learning and overall service-learning outcomes. Table 1.1 includes a summary of essential service-learning elements that have been described in the literature, including academic content connections, active reflection, authentic community needs, development, diversity, meaningful service, reciprocity, and student voice (e.g., Berger

Kaye, 2004; Campus Compact, 2007; Eyler & Giles, 1994, 1999; Mintz & Hesser, 1996; University of Central Florida, 2011). In this section, we will examine each of these elements with some of the elements contextualized by the service-learning project examples presented earlier in this chapter; you will note how the absence of any of these elements would transform the described activities into something other than service-learning.

Table 1.1
Summary of Essential Elements of Service-Learning

Element	Brief Description
Academic Content Connections	Service activities are conducted in the context of course objectives. In other words, service-learning involves integrated learning in which content knowledge and skills inform related service activities and then service activities in turn enhance course content.
Active Reflection	Intentional, systematic reflection of experience must take place in order to thoughtfully connect service-learning experiences with the targeted curriculum.
Authentic Community Needs	Community may be defined locally, regionally, nationally, or globally, but the identified needs being targeted through service activities must be authentically identified, recognized, valued, and unmet.
Development	Service-learning can occur in different ways at different stages. Students may be involved in activities that educate, service, enable, or empower and they may observe, participate, or provide leadership in the process.

Element	Brief Description
Diversity	A broad cross-section of students working in diverse settings with diverse populations is exposed to new and varied issues and activities across communities.
Meaningful Service	Service tasks need to be worthwhile and challenging in order to strengthen students' critical thinking and foster civic responsibility while improving communities.
Reciprocity	The service and learning must be worthwhile for both the student and the community. There must be reciprocity between those providing the service and those served. True partnerships, collaborations, and shared responsibilities are inherent in this element.
Student Voice	Students must take ownership and direct their own learning as well as the benefits of their work experienced in the community. Decision making and responsibility influence this element.

Academic Content Connections. As indicated in Table 1.1, close connections to academic content afford integrated learning in which content knowledge and skills inform related service activities and then service activities in turn enhance course content. To illustrate this element, consider the possibility of students participating in many of the activities within the service-learning project examples described earlier in this chapter without the context of course objectives. For example, university students might volunteer to help with a parent support group for children who are deaf or hard of hearing. However, providing babysitting services or helping with coffee hour would provide very different experiences than providing indirect aural habilitation intervention services within the context of a parent workshop. In this project example, the academic course work is critical to the development of the necessary knowledge and/or skills to ensure adequate preparation for completion of the described aural habilitation service activities.

Active Reflection. Intentional, active, and ongoing active reflection often has been identified as the element that can transform simple experiences into learning. For example, without engaging in ongoing reflection on connections between information learned about types of chemotherapy and specifics like length of treatment and side effects, it would be possible for the students managing the previously described fundraiser project to have outcomes that were inadequate to meet the actual needs of the identified patients. Although it might be fine to raise enough money for a child in a developing country to pay for a specific type of chemotherapy, this act may not result in a positive outcome if financial support is not provided for transportation to a facility offering this type of treatment or if funds are available for only a very brief round of treatment in the case of a specific cancer that has been proven to require lengthy chemotherapy protocols. Critical reflection activities may include discussion assignments, interviews, journaling, analytic papers, portfolios, reading responses, or presentations (e.g., Hurd, 2007).

Authentic Community Needs. Similarly, it would be possible for college students to administer developmental screenings for children who are already enrolled in an afterschool program for children who are gifted. However, it is unlikely that this activity would address a recognized need for the community in general, or even for the identified children in particular, since they already would have undergone extensive developmental and academic testing to be identified for a gifted program. This illustrates a clear contrast to college students administering developmental screenings for children in a homeless shelter who most likely would be receiving very limited or inconsistent health and/or educational services; performing screenings in this case would address a recognized need for "at-risk" children.

Development. Service-learning activities may involve any level of development, which could include educating, providing services, enabling, and/or empowering. Although the students in the chemotherapy project example did not have the ability to provide the required services, they were able to empower the individuals in need to obtain the relevant services. You likely can see how providing information on relevant chemotherapy services would have accomplished development at a different level.

Diversity. Diversity is inherent in service-learning as a broad cross-section of students working in diverse settings with diverse populations is exposed to new and varied issues and activities across communities. In identifying authentic community needs, students often are exposed to diverse populations to which they may not have been exposed otherwise. These types of experiences can have long-range effects on how students consider the possible impact of their actions on a wide range of individuals.

Meaningful Service. Although "meaningful" may have different connotations for different people, there is a shared understanding of significance and impact underlying most definitions or beliefs associated with the concept of "meaningful." With respect to service-learning, it is possible to take action in a given community without that action having any notable impact on anyone. Consider for example, the previously described project in which the preschool students grew vegetables and then donated the crops to a local soup kitchen. What if the soup kitchen did not have a way to cook vegetables for its clients? The students would still be providing a service, but the meaning or impact would be different.

Reciprocity. Service-learning is a reciprocal process that should involve faculty members, students, and the community. In order for true reciprocity to exist, there must be benefits for both those providing the services (i.e., students directly and faculty members indirectly) and those receiving the services (i.e., community agencies/organizations and members). It is not sufficient for students to practice or apply what they are learning in a course for the sake of gaining experience; the practice or application must provide a direct benefit to the community. The partnership and collaboration strategies typically involved in service-learning naturally support ongoing positive community connections that yield reciprocity. To illustrate this concept, we can think back to the earlier example where the graduate speech–language pathology students partnered with a parent support group to prepare and offer family workshops on aural habilitation techniques. If the parent support group had participated in a similar workshop the month prior, it could be argued that it was only the students who benefitted from providing the workshop by gaining this type of clinical experience.

Student Voice. Although one could argue that students should be actively engaged in all academic activities, service-learning provides unique opportunities for students to take ownership in shaping the direction of their own learning and the benefits of their work experienced in the community. Students often are able to select, design, implement, and evaluate various components of their service activities, which can encourage relevancy and sustained interest.

In summary, service-learning can offer students unique learning opportunities in real-world contexts. In this chapter, we examined a number of key considerations and elements that must be taken into account when planning and executing service-learning projects in general. In Chapter 2, we will turn our attention to some specific considerations for service-learning in the context of speech–language pathology (SLP) and audiology.

2

SL in Communication Sciences and Disorders

There is a growing body of literature that supports the efficacy of service-learning as a pedagogical tool in higher education. Service-learning has been reported to have a positive impact on student: (a) academic learning (e.g., Astin & Sax, 1998); (b) application of course-related knowledge and skills (e.g., Balazadeh, 1996); (c) communication and leadership skills (e.g., Vogelgesang & Astin, 2000); (d) understanding of cultural, racial, and individual differences (e.g., Myers-Lipton, 1996); (e) social responsibility (e.g., Kendrick, 1996); and (f) demonstrated complexity of understanding, problem solving, and critical thinking (e.g., Batchelder & Root, 1994). Considering the relevance of these positive outcomes to higher education in general and communication sciences and disorders in particular, service-learning presents itself as a potentially powerful model for instruction. However, there is a lack of documentation on the efficacy of service-learning in our field and a lack of literature to guide students and faculty in the practicalities of conducting service-learning.

A Service-Learning Project Model for Communication Sciences and Disorders

In this chapter, we will review a proposed service-learning project model that is tailored to the fields of speech–language pathology and audiology specifically. The model proposed in this chapter draws from a variety of service-learning models that have been presented in a range of other fields (e.g., Bowdon, 2005; University of Minnesota, 2011) and includes several categories and sub-categories of service-learning projects that are relevant to our field in particular. Table 2.1 identifies the two major categories of service-learning projects within the proposed service-learning project model as follows: (a) Practice-Oriented Projects and (b) Policy-Oriented Projects. The foci and sub-categories within these two categories are detailed below.

Table 2.1

Service-Learning Project Model for Communication Sciences and Disorders

Category	Focus	Sub-Categories
Practice-Oriented Projects	Direct Service Focus	• People-Oriented • Product-Oriented • Education-Oriented
	Indirect Service Focus	• Research • Community Building/ Organization
Policy-Oriented Projects	Research Focus	
	Advocacy/ Activism Focus	

Practice-Oriented Projects

Given the clinical nature of the fields of speech–language pathology and audiology, many service-learning projects fall within this category. As you know, "clinical" work encompasses a wide range of activities since speech–language pathologists and audiologists provide services to prevent, diagnose, evaluate, and treat communication disorders (American Speech-Language-Hearing Association, 2011b). Therefore, service-learning projects can offer students opportunities to gain a wide range of clinically related experiences in our fields. The following sub-categories within the major category of Practice-Oriented Projects help to specify the varying foci of service-learned projects within this category: (a) Direct-Service-Focused Projects, including People-Oriented, Product-Oriented, and Education-Oriented Projects, and (b) Indirect-Service-Focused Projects, including Research and Community-Oriented Projects.

Direct-Service-Focused Projects. With this type of service-learning project, students work directly with consumers, clients, patients, and/or staff to meet a specified community need. This may be the category you first thought about when you started reading this chapter. You may have envisioned yourself having the opportunity to provide speech, language, or hearing intervention services. These types of projects can be further specified within the subcategories of (a) people-oriented projects, (b) product-oriented projects, and (c) education-oriented projects. Let's consider some examples in each of these sub-categories.

In the case of a people-oriented service-learning project, students work directly with consumers, clients, patients, and/or staff to provide a needed service. As in the following examples, these types of service-focused projects may involve prevention, diagnosis, or treatment of a speech, language, or hearing issue: (a) students in a language disorders class work with children in a preschool for disadvantaged children to build vocabulary skills, (b) students in an audiology class perform hearing screenings for Head Start children, and (c) a student in an augmentative and alternative communication (AAC) class targets social goals with a young girl using AAC in the context of Girl Scout meetings.

When completing a product-focused project, students create a product for a community agency or its consumers, clients, patients, and/or staff. One example of this type of project could involve students in an American Sign Language (ASL) class developing a training manual to be used within an ASL instructional course that they facilitate for a local support group for parents of children with hearing impairments. In this example, the training manual is the "product," which ends up being used clinically.

Finally, when completing education-focused service-learning projects, students educate community members about communication-related issues. Students may educate the public at large or specific sub-groups of the community on broader issues relating to the nature of communication and/or the profession. Additionally, they may focus their education efforts on more specific issues like speech, language, hearing, and related disorders/ disabilities along with related services and providers. The following project example includes a narrow focus on stuttering as a communication disorders specifically. Students in a fluency class prepare and deliver a presentation on the nature and treatment of fluency disorders for the teachers in a school that has several enrolled children who stutter.

Indirect-Service-Focused Projects. In contrast to the above descriptions and examples of direct-service-focused projects, students working on indirect-service-focused projects do not participate in direct service delivery. These types of projects most often fall into the categories of research or community building. Students may think of themselves as being more "behind the scenes" when working on these types of projects.

Research-oriented projects may be informal, such as in the example of students in a voice and resonance disorders class conducting research on all facilities offering voice care services in a given community. In the case of this project, individuals in a particular geographic location will benefit from the directory of services that is generated. In contrast, research-oriented projects can have far-reaching effects if they are more formalized as in examples where students complete systematic reviews or meta-analyses that eventually get published in peer-reviewed journals and/or presented at professional conferences. Students in a feeding and swallowing course might complete a systematic review of all interventions for a specified type of feeding disorder to inform the protocols of a feeding/swallowing team in a given medical facility. However, the outcome of this review has relevance to all researchers and clinicians practicing in this area; therefore, wide dissemination through presentation and publication is an important outcome for this type of project.

Community-building or organizing-oriented projects afford students opportunities to advance community issues. Examples range from projects at the local level where students institute new community organizations to projects where community building is facilitated at the national level. There are many organizations that exist at the national level (e.g., United Cerebral Palsy, Down Syndrome Congress) and also have chapters at the local or regional level designed to be more direct-service oriented. Service-learning projects within organizations such as these can give students new perspective on sub-communities within the larger disability community.

Policy-Oriented Projects

Although students often primarily focus on the more clinical aspects of speech–language pathology and audiology (i.e., the "micro" level), we must also recall that policies provide critical underpinnings for service delivery. If there are no policies in place to ensure that clients with communication disorders have rights to access speech, language, and hearing services, there will be a dramatic change in the clinical landscape. Therefore, students working on policy-oriented service-learning projects may have very real opportunities to affect our fields at a more "macro" level. The following sub-categories within the major category of practice-oriented projects provide additional specificity for service-learning projects within this category: (a) direct-service-focused projects, including people-oriented, product-oriented, and education-oriented projects, and (b) indirect-service-focused projects, including research and community-oriented projects.

Research Focus. With this type of service-learning project, students engage in assessing and developing ideas for developing the field or community in a specified area. One example of a project that might fall in this category would be a group of students conducting a survey for a community-based clinic providing low-cost or free communication assessments and interventions for elderly clients. Via the survey, the students could assist the community-based clinic in identifying barriers to senior citizens accessing services and possibly even identifying supports that allow these potential clients to overcome these barriers. From there, the clinic could make decisions about new or altered policies that would be more supportive of clients accessing needed services.

Advocacy/Activism Focus. Focused advocacy is sometimes necessary to make meaningful changes in our field. The American Speech-Language-Hearing Association, which is the professional, scientific, and credentialing association for speech–language pathologists, audiologists, and related scientists in the United States, and state-level professional organizations have public policy agendas designed to protect the rights of individuals with communication disabilities and those who practice or conduct research in our fields. These agendas often include policy, funding, and personnel priorities, and students may become involved in the development or activism surrounding these priorities (e.g., American Speech-Language-Hearing Association, 2011a). Additionally, disability-specific organizations such as those mentioned previously often get involved in lobbying or activism related to the rights and the services of individuals with communication disorders. Again, service-learning projects in this area have the potential to yield widespread impact for individuals with disabilities.

One example of this is in the area of AAC. It is only since the year 2000 that all Medicaid programs in the United States have been providing coverage of AAC devices. This milestone required tireless advocacy and lobbying on the part of various professionals and organizations over many years. This advocacy was well worth it since it ended up yielding access to communication for a group of individuals with critical needs and also influenced coverage of AAC devices by other groups of individuals relying on other third-party funding sources (e.g., Medicare, private health insurance, special education, early intervention, vocational rehabilitation). The need for advocacy in this area continues since universal coverage of AAC devices is still not available.

In conclusion, service-learning falls in line with the philosophy that "variety is the spice of life!" There are many types of service-learning projects that can be tailored to be relevant to the course content in any number of speech–language pathology and audiology classes. Similarly, there is no shortage of opportunities for students to exert initiative in identifying and/or developing service-learning projects that are responsive to their own interests.

3

KEY PLAYERS AND COMMON SL EXPECTATIONS

Now that you have considered the relevance of service-learning to communication sciences and disorders as a field, let's examine the key players in the service-learning process, including students, community partner personnel, and faculty members. When involved in a service-learning project, it is important for students to realize that they are not the only ones who come to the table (or to the project in this case) with expectations! Community partners involved in the project and faculty members facilitating the service-learning experience will inevitably have expectations with respect to how the project will progress and what the related benefits of the project might be.

Students

Much has been written about students' perceptions of the benefits of service-learning upon project completion, but less is known about students' perceptions of service-learning prior to engaging in the process. As the key learner and service provider within the context of a service-learning project, the student carries a good deal of responsibility. After all, service-learning falls within the construct of "active" learning, so at the very least, you will come to the table with the notion that you will be actively engaged in your service-learning class.

Student expectations may vary based on personality traits, learning style, knowledge and skill base, and past experience. Therefore, a given expectation may excite one student and cause another student to be anxious prior to starting a service-learning project. However, it is important to remember that all types of students can benefit from involvement in service-learning projects. Which of the following common service-learning expectations are exciting from your perspective?

- Opportunity to apply course content.
- Opportunity to build your "resume" or differentiate your education from that of others.
- Opportunity to collaborate with others.
- Opportunity to develop communication skills.
- Opportunity to gain a deeper understanding of a given community and associated issues (could be a local, state, national, or global community).
- Opportunity to gain leadership experience.
- Opportunity to gain "real-world" experience.
- Opportunity to learn by "doing."
- Opportunity to network more widely.
- Opportunity to problem-solve.
- Opportunity to "rise to a challenge."

Even if some of the above-listed opportunities are new or even somewhat intimidating for you, it would be difficult to argue that they would not ultimately benefit you. The likelihood that you will gain meaningful new knowledge and skills and perhaps even gain a deeper awareness of civic responsibility and/or moral character often seems to be magnified in the context of a service-learning course.

Furthermore, although students take on significant responsibility through service-learning in responding to the types of opportunities listed above, this responsibility fits within the safe and supervised context of the course. In addition to having university professors as resources, students taking service-learning courses also have access to the additional field-related resources through the community partners with whom they are assigned to work, which brings us to this next group of key players in the service-learning process.

Community Partner Personnel

In the fields of speech–language pathology and audiology, there is a wealth of potential community partners for service-learning projects. Students may contract to work with such entities as public schools or school districts, disability-specific associations or foundations (e.g., United Cerebral Palsy), government-funded service programs (e.g., Head Start), support groups (e.g., Hands & Voices), or funding agencies (e.g., Medicaid). To give you an idea of the variety of options that exist for community partners in our field, even the list of agencies with whom my own students have partnered to date would be too long to list here. No matter which agencies students partner with, service-learning projects present ideal opportunities for university students and community partner personnel to actively engage within the community and move away from the "ivory tower" approach to teaching and conducting research.

Some potential expectations on the part of partnering agency personnel are listed below.

- Opportunity to access relevant expertise and resources.
- Opportunity to gain assistance in meeting critical agency needs.
- Opportunity to generate new ideas and energy.
- Opportunity to make personal connections with university students and personnel.
- Opportunity to work with knowledgeable and skilled students.

Some community agencies have a long history of engagement with university communities, whereas others may have no history of collaborating with university students, faculties, or programs. This means that there may be a great deal of variability in the way different community partner personnel approach the practical aspects of participating in a service-learning project. Table 3.1 represents two ends of the spectrum with respect to community agency expectations.

Table 3.1
Examples of Community Agency Expectations for Service-Learning

Activity	Clearly Defined Service-Learning Activities and Expectations	Open-Ended Service-Learning Activities and Expectations
Defining the Project	Initiate the project by presenting a clear and concise description of the project itself or the agency need.	Initiate the project with limited details on the project or agency need.
Identifying Agency Contacts	Assign one consistent contact for students throughout the duration of the project.	Assign no specific contact for students or repeatedly change the assigned contact throughout the project.
Project Meetings	Hold regularly scheduled meetings to ensure ongoing contact.	Maintain no meeting schedule and limited contact.
Project Milestones	Identify clear project milestones or check-points for the project.	Identify no project milestones and/or very limited feedback throughout the project.
Instructor Input	Request regular or significant instructor input.	Request very little instructor input.

Although you may initially think that you would not want to be in the bad position of being assigned to work with an agency that approached a service-learning project as described in the last column of the above table, it is important to go back to the reciprocal relationship we discussed in Chapter 2. As a key player in service-learning, you are able to contribute to all aspects of the service-learning project—even the procedural aspects. We will review helpful procedures for students to follow when conducting service-learning projects in the next chapter, so you will have some tools in your service-learning toolkits to deal with some of the above-listed issues. Furthermore, it is important to recall that partnering agency personnel often are stretched very thin with respect to their own work. Therefore, it is not typically the case that agency doesn't value the service-learning project; rather, it may be the reality that additional activities associated with the project do not work well within the confines of an already tight schedule with limited resources, as is the case for many nonprofit agencies in current times, for example.

University Faculty Members / Course Instructors

Just because many activities involved in service-learning projects take place off campus, it doesn't mean that the university faculty member or the instructor teaching your course is not a key player in the service-learning process. If a service-learning project is part of your class, the odds are that it was your instructor who made the decision to include this type of learning experience in the course in the first place. At the very least, the instructor should have had the opportunity to provide at least some input into the project even if the course was designed by someone else.

Since service-learning is closely tied to course objectives, the course instructor will be responsible for ensuring that relevant content is covered via non-service-learning course components. These course components may include activities such as lectures, web-based modules, workshops, readings, lab experiences, and simulations. Additionally, it is likely that the instructor will assess your learning through a variety of mechanisms outside the service-learning project. A service-learning course also will often include more traditional forms of assessment like exams, written assignments, and class presentations, for example.

Just as partnering agency personnel will operate in environments that will vary in terms of the resources and supports to which they have access, the same can be said for course instructors. Some instructors may teach in environments where service-learning has been institutionalized and there may be entire offices dedicated to service-learning in particular or to experiential learning more generally. In these institutions, it is likely that course instructors have access to staff members who can assist in preparing for and teaching service-learning classes. It may even be the case that the institution provides guidelines or requirements for classes to be designated as official "service-learning" classes. See Table 3.2 for a checklist adapted from the criteria in place for service-learning course designation at the University of Central Florida (2007).

At the other extreme, some course instructors may teach in institutions that may somewhat value experiential learning, but do not provide supports for service-learning activities or courses. In these cases, it is still possible to have innovative instructors who are very skilled at managing service-learning course components. Again, in either case, the suggestions provided in the next chapter can go a long way in helping to ensure that everyone has a successful service-learning experience.

Table 3.2

Sample Criteria Evaluation Tool for SL Course or Syllabus

Criteria for Described Service-Learning Assignment	Criteria Met or Not Met?		Description/Notes
Addresses an authentic need in the community at a campus, local, regional, or global level.	Met	Not Met	
Addresses one or more course objectives.	Met	Not Met	
Demonstrates clear connections to course content.	Met	Not Met	

Criteria for Described Service-Learning Assignment	Criteria Met or Not Met?		Description/Notes
Involves reciprocity between course and community.	Met	Not Met	
Involves a minimum of 15 hours of student service.	Met	Not Met	
Involves structured reflections.	Met	Not Met	
Partnering community agency is a nonprofit or governmental agency (e.g., public school, philanthropic arm of for-profit organization).	Met	Not Met	
All students in the course are required to complete service-learning activities.	Met	Not Met	
A grade is assigned for achievement of course objectives via SL.	Met	Not Met	

4

EVIDENCE OF LEARNING: SAMPLE SL PROJECT

Now that we have reviewed some common categories of service-learning projects in speech–language pathology and audiology and considered some general examples of projects within each category, we will turn our attention to a more detailed service-learning project example. This project is presented in the context of a research study that was conducted to determine the effects on several key players involved in the project. The project is described with a level of detail that will allow you to consider the project from the perspectives of the various stakeholders discussed in Chapter 2 and as a prelude to the model service-learning components and procedures that will be presented in Chapter 5. It should be noted that preliminary results for this research study originally were presented at the Annual Convention of the American Speech–language-Hearing Association in San Diego, CA (Kent-Walsh, 2005).

Detailed Service-Learning Project Example: *TeenTech*

Service-Learning Project Background. The American Speech–Language-Hearing Association (2005) defines augmentative and alternative communication (AAC) as follows:

> *Augmentative and alternative communication (AAC) refers to an area of research, clinical, and educational practice. AAC involves attempts to study and when necessary compensate for temporary or permanent impairments, activity limitations, and participation restrictions of individuals with severe disorders of speech–language production and/or comprehension, including spoken and written modes of communication.*
> (p. 413)

AAC falls under a broader category of assistive technology (AT), which includes any type of technology that a person might use to compensate for a disability or impairment. It can include no-tech communication options (e.g., communication boards and books), low/mid-tech devices (e.g., voice output devices with recorded speech), or high-tech devices (e.g., computerized voice-output devices with synthesized speech) (Binger & Kent-Walsh, 2010). ASHA includes AAC and AT within one of the nine categories in which graduate speech–language pathology students are required to demonstrate knowledge and skills as delineated in the Standards for the Certificate of Clinical Competence (American-Speech-Language-Hearing Association, 2005). However, undergraduate students often do not have opportunities to take coursework or gain clinical experience in this area. The project described in this example comprised a unique opportunity for undergraduate students to work with individuals who use AAC in the context of an elective course in AAC that involved a service-learning requirement.

Service-Learning Project Overview. All students taking the referenced undergraduate class in AAC completed the same service-learning project—they served as facilitators for middle school students with AAC/AT needs who were participating in a day camp program designed to facilitate the use of AAC/AT within educational activities. *TeenTech* was a week-long curriculum-based summer day camp for middle school students with disabilities and their parents, caregivers, and/or educators that took place on campus at the University of Central Florida in Orlando. The mission of the *TeenTech* program was to have undergraduate students work collaboratively with participating campers to identify and learn to use various hardware and software solutions to enhance camper participation in educational activities in the long term.

Purpose and Research Objectives. A research study was designed and executed to evaluate the effects of undergraduate student service-learning activities within the day-camp program for middle and high school students with AAC/AT needs on:

- The participating undergraduate service-learning students' perceived learning related to AAC/AT technology.
- The participating undergraduate service-learning students' perceived learning related to clients with AAC/AT needs.
- The participating middle and high school students' perceived AAC/AT technology skills.
- The participating parents' satisfaction with the day-camp program.
- The community partner personnel's satisfaction with undergraduate service-learning student contributions to the *TeenTech* program and work with participating middle and high school students.

Participants and Program Description. Sixteen undergraduate students (15 females, 1 male; age range = 20 – 50 years) enrolled in an undergraduate class in AAC participated as *TeenTech* facilitators. Fifteen students with developmental disabilities (8 females, 7 males; age range = 11 – 21 years) participated in the *TeenTech* program as campers. Prior to the beginning of camp and in coordination with relevant content presented in class, the *TeenTech* facilitators participated in an intensive three-day hardware and software training to develop knowledge and skills of various AAC/AT options that would be relevant to the needs of the campers.

The theme for the *TeenTech* curriculum was African animals. Each day, participants worked with the undergraduate student facilitators to learn to use new hardware and software and/or to more effectively use hardware and software with which they had prior familiarity. Activities centered on literacy and math constructs with the ultimate goal of each student completing a written report on an African animal of choice. Students did Internet and field-based research (at Walt Disney World's Animal Kingdom) for their reports. On the final day of *TeenTech,* all participants delivered their reports to an audience of approximately 40 students, family members, and professionals.

Descriptive and Qualitative Research Methodology. In addition to completing formative and summative written reflections, the service-learning student facilitators completed pre- and post-participation Likert scale questionnaires to rate their perceived knowledge and skills related to (a) AAC/AT and (b) working with children with AAC/AT needs, before and after the service-learning training and activities associated with *TeenTech*. Similarly, the participating middle school students completed pre- and post-participation questionnaires to rate their perceived knowledge and ease of use with various AAC/AT options for use in academic contexts. The parents whose children participated in *TeenTech* and the sponsoring agency supervisors completed post-participation questionnaires to gauge their satisfaction with the work of the service-learning student facilitators. The below two 5-point Likert scale questionnaires were used for the AAC/AT client-related items and technology-related items respectively on the service-learning student facilitator questionnaires.

Table 4.1

Likert Scale Used for Client-Related Service-Learning Student Facilitator Pre- and Post-Participation Questionnaire Items

Not At All Knowledgeable	Somewhat Knowledgeable	Knowledgeable	Very Knowledgeable	Expert Clinician or Educator
1	2	3	4	5

Table 4.2

Likert Scale Used for Technology-Related Service-Learning Student Facilitator Pre- and Post-Participation Questionnaire Items

Not At All Familiar	Somewhat Familiar	Familiar	Very Familiar	Expert User
(i.e., I do not recognize the name or only recognize the name of the AAC/AT option)	(i.e., I recognize the name and know the purpose of the AAC/AT option)	(i.e., I know the name of the AAC/AT option and some of its key features)	(i.e., I know how to operate/use some of the functions of the AAC/AT option)	(i.e., I feel relatively confident when operating/using this AAC/AT option)
1	2	3	4	5

Summary of Results. Table 4.3 summarizes the results of the findings related to the *TeenTech* program. In general, the results indicate a high level of satisfaction expressed by all key players. Additionally, the participating student facilitators showed statistically significant increases in their perceived levels of knowledge and skill related to clients with AAC/AT needs and AAC/AT technology.

Table 4.3

Summary of Results for *TeenTech* Outcome Study

Service-Learning Student Facilitators	Participating Middle School Students	Parents of Participating Middle School Students	Sponsoring Agency Supervisors
Statistically significant increases in students' perceived learning across all questions related to AAC/AT clients and technology (p < .001). • Average Perceived AAC/AT Client Knowledge/Skill *Pre-SL Average* Perceived AAC/AT Client Knowledge/Skill *Post-SL Average* = 1.1 : 3.6 • Average Perceived AAC/AT Technology Knowledge/Skill *Pre-SL Average* Perceived AAC/AT Technology Knowledge/Skill *Post-SL Average* = 1.5 : 3.1	Noted increases in student knowledge and skills. • 93% of students perceived that: (a) they learned at least one new thing that was relevant to them related to personal use of AAC/AT tools and (b) they learned new information related to African Animals during their participation in *TeenTech.*	Noted parent satisfaction. • 100% of parents indicated that *TeenTech* and the service-learning student interns met their children's needs and benefited their children. • Inductive qualitative analyses (Boyatzis, 1998) of participating parents' written feedback revealed the following themes: (a) value of interaction with facilitators and peers, (b) value of using AAC/AT during community activities, and (c) value of learning how to use new AAC/AT tools.	Noted supervisor satisfaction. • 100% of student service-learning facilitators received the highest possible satisfaction rating. • Supervisors indicated interns worked very effectively with the participating clients and families and were highly effective in their application of AAC/AT tools with clients.
Noted high student satisfaction with service-learning experiences. • Inductive qualitative analyses of written reflections (Boyatzis, 1998) indicated that student satisfaction related to the following themes: intensive training component, authentic hands-on application with clients, rewarding nature and overall value of service-learning activities.			

Discussion. In addition to anecdotal reports of the efficacy of service-learning in communication sciences and disorders (e.g., Scherz, 2008), published reports of outcomes are beginning to emerge in the literature (e.g., Bailey & Angell, 2005; Goldberg, Richburg & Wood, 2008). As researchers continue to effectively document the value of service-learning, it is likely that additional faculty and students will experience its value in their courses (e.g., Eyler, Giles, Stenson & Gray, 2001; Steinberg, Bringle & Williams, 2010). The service-learning project and associated data presented in this chapter offer early indications of the value of service-learning and should provide you with some ideas as to the type of benefits you may experience when participating in service-learning activities.

5

MODEL SL PROJECT COMPONENTS AND PROCEDURES

After considering an example of a service-learning project that yielded positive outcomes, you may be optimistic about the prospect of completing a service-learning project that is of particular interest to you. However, effective service-learning does not magically happen on its own! In order to help you enjoy a successful service-learning experience, this chapter will describe some suggested steps that you can take to keep your project running smoothly. We will first consider four stages of the service-learning process and then look at a number of tools that can help you to effectively and efficiently manage the range of agency and course expectations that you may encounter.

Service-Learning Project Stages

Cathryn Berger Kaye (2004) suggested that the service-learning process can be broken into four stages: (a) *preparation*, (b) *action*, (c) *demonstration*, and (d) *reflection*. Formally or informally approaching a service-learning project with these four stages in mind can assist students in planning to effectively execute all necessary service-learning activities. Berger Kaye's suggested stages have been summarized and adapted in this section for application in university courses in communication sciences and disorders.

Preparation: During the *preparation* stage, students start by identifying a specific need in the community and move to the point of being ready to begin to address the need through a well-defined service-learning project. This stage typically involves (a) conducting research, (b) drawing on knowledge and skills previously acquired and those relevant to the academic course in progress, (c) collaborating with the partnering community agency, and (d) specifically defining realistic parameters for the project.

Action: Once students are ready to begin their projects, they move into the *action* stage. This stage may involve direct service, indirect service, research, and/or advocacy as covered in Chapter 2. In other words, this is the "doing" stage; students are actively involved in the work at hand.

Demonstration: The *demonstration* stage comes into play at the end of the project when students demonstrate their skills, knowledge, insights, and outcomes of the service-learning project. This demonstration may take place in the context of the partnering agency (e.g., delivering a workshop for teachers of children with language disorders), within the context of the academic course (e.g., delivering a presentation to the course instructor and classmates to report on the process and outcomes of the service-learning project), or even in a broader community context (e.g., distributing flyers on hearing loss prevention to families of children attending an elementary school). In general, demonstration could include activities such as reports, presentations, and publications.

Reflection: The fourth and final stage of the service-learning process, *reflection,* actually runs for the duration of the service-learning project. Through systematic reflection, students examine their plans and experiences and reshape the direction of their service-learning activities as they obtain input from course instructors and partnering agency contacts. In some cases, instructors provide specific prompts for discussion assignments and in other cases, students are asked to keep a more informal journal or log of experiences over time. In either case, the key is for students to try to sort out reports of what actually happened from how things made them feel (e.g., Berger Kaye, 2004). Given the strong emotional reactions that students often have when working with "real people" for the first time in a professional context, it is sometimes easiest for students to use a format that allows them to (a) describe what happened, (b) discuss thoughts and related feelings,

(c) make connections to course objectives, and then (d) consider any feedback that should be obtained and/or how the next steps in the project should take shape.

Suggested Tools for Successful Service-Learning Projects

Although some course instructors provide specific tools (e.g., forms, contracts) that students *must* use as they move through the above-described stages of their service-learning projects, other instructors may ask students to develop or customize their own documentation. This section includes practical suggestions for tools that can help students maintain consistent and accurate documentation for service-learning projects. You should note that examples of suggested tools and forms that may be helpful as you complete your service-learning activities are included in the appendices.

Service-Learning Project Descriptions. Although some course instructors provide specific service-learning project options from which students can choose, other instructors may provide students with the option to suggest and develop their own service-learning projects. If you encounter the latter option, you will be in the unique position of being able to tailor a project around your own interests and contacts. However, there are several factors you should keep in mind when proposing a project.

First and foremost, it is always a good idea to keep a variation of the proverbial KISS philosophy in mind—"keep it simple and straightforward." Sometimes students get so excited about the possibilities when planning projects that they overestimate what they can accomplish within a semester or a portion of a semester. However, most course instructors and agency representatives will agree that it is far better to propose something that can be accomplished with good quality than to propose something more elaborate that may not get completed or that may not be up to par in the end. Therefore, it is important to keep the scope of the project and the project time line reasonable for everyone involved. Even if you are willing to devote a great deal of concentrated time and effort to various aspects of your project, you must remember that agency representatives and course instructors need to be given adequate time to provide feedback and to complete any aspects of the project for which they must take responsibility. Since these individuals typically have numerous projects and deadlines on their plates at any given time, they also will need to determine if the project is doable from their perspectives.

Appendix A contains a document with sample service-learning project descriptions. You will see that the entries for each project contain enough information for students and course instructors to determine the general scope and requirements of the project as well as information relative to the partnering agencies. When submitting this type of brief project proposal to a course instructor, it is suggested that you include the name of the partnering agency, contact information for the agency, and any unique project requirements of which you may be aware (e.g., background check requirements to be on site, required experience, or timelines). Of course, the most important aspect of your proposal will be a brief description of the project goals and/or the activities that will be associated with completion of the project. Although instructors typically do not require detailed project information when students submit project proposals, it is important to give your instructors at least enough information for them to determine the relevance of the project to the course objectives.

Service-Learning Project Contract. After you have either selected a project or had a proposed project approved, you will need to move into a more detailed planning phase. Even if your course instructor does not require the completion of a specific Service-Learning Project Contract (see Appendix B for sample), it is a good idea to complete this type of document to ensure that all key players are on the same page so to speak. Things will go more smoothly for you if there is a shared understanding between you, your course instructor, and your community partner contact as to how your project will be completed.

The sample contract in Appendix B is structured to yield a reference document that the student, course instructor, and community partner personnel can follow throughout the semester once the document has been finalized. Therefore, this sample document will be used as a guide to discuss key elements of a *Service-Learning Project Contract* in this section. The first section of the document contains contact details for each of the individuals involved in the project as well as logistical details such as expected project start/end dates and the approximate number of hours to be completed on the project. It should be noted that weekly hour expectations may involve on-site activities completed on specified days/times (e.g., service-delivery at the agency's facility) and/or other activities to be completed at the location and time chosen by the student (e.g., library or web-based research); in either case, these expectations should be explicitly discussed and documented prior to initiation of the project.

The second section of the sample contract includes two key elements that typically are completed collaboratively by the student and a partnering agency representative: (a) the detailed service-learning project description, and (b) the detailed project timeline. The project description affords the student and partner agency personnel the opportunity to specify additional details beyond the general description that may have been generated when the project was initially conceived. After the project description, the timeline is perhaps the most important aspect of the contract since it allows everyone to closely monitor the project progress and outcomes to ensure timely completion of all required activities. The sample timeline within the contract provided in Appendix B includes a "Deadline" column with space to input the agreed upon dates and a "Latest Date" listing for each project milestone. The "Latest Date" may or may not be specified by the course instructor. The course instructor may wish to communicate the latest dates by which certain project milestones should be completed to ensure coordination with content being covered in the course or to ensure adequate time to provide students with feedback. You may be well advised to seek input from your course instructor before confirming deadlines with your agency contact person.

The final section of the sample project contract in Appendix B contains information on suggested guidelines and limitations to which students, community partner personnel, and course instructors can formally agree. This information helps everyone to clearly know their responsibilities and rights in order to conduct themselves responsibly on a project. Just as it is important for students to uphold their responsibilities, it also is important for students to know whom they can contact in cases where they experience difficulties or have questions. In laying out these things explicitly in the contract, students can feel comfortable in knowing how to proceed in any number of situations.

Service-Learning Hour Log. Another way to consistently document your work on your service-learning project is to keep an hour log throughout the duration of your project. Even if this is not formally required by your course instructor or agency contact, it can provide additional documentation on the process of developing your project when you submit or execute your finalized project. In some cases, course instructors or agency contacts assign work that they think will not take long to complete, but they can then be surprised when students submit documentation for the work that went into completing individual project milestones. The more detail you provide when completing an hour log such as the sample provided in Appendix C, the better.

Weekly Service-Learning Reflection Tool. As previously mentioned, it is sometimes challenging for students to sort out their reflections on service-learning activities even when there is a specific reflection prompt to be considered. Therefore, students may want to consider using a tool that helps them organize their thoughts, reflections, and feelings. As suggested by other service-learning practitioners (e.g., Berger Kay, 2004), the reflection tool provided in Appendix D guides students in recording service-learning activities, reactions, connections to course content, and next steps. This tool may be used as the sole reflection product or it may be used to assist in formulating responses to more specific reflection prompts provided by course instructors, for example.

Evaluation Forms. Appendices E and F provide samples of evaluation forms that can be used to document project feedback from agency contacts and students. Forms such as these may directly lead to the formulation of part of the grade for your service-learning project or they may play a more informal role in the evaluation process. Either way, these forms can provide the course instructor with valuable information on the process of project completion and on the overall value of the completed project. It is often fascinating for students to receive feedback from the real world via agency contacts and peers. Students frequently state that this type of feedback really helps to put things into perspective for them.

After reviewing the suggested forms and contracts in this chapter and the accompanying samples in the Appendices, you may be left with the feeling that you can never plan too much when executing a service-learning project. This is typically an accurate assessment! While service-learning projects are incredibly valuable and often yield some of the most seminal experiences of students' academic careers, they also are incredibly involved. As Beth Mabry (1998) argued, "time, contact, and reflection matter" (p. 32) when it comes to service-learning and student outcomes! Therefore, an investment in systematic planning and execution should return worthwhile dividends.

Wrap-Up

Hopefully this book has piqued your interest in service-learning and provided you with an overview of the nature of service-learning as well as practical aspects of completing service-learning projects. As a faculty member in communication sciences and disorders who has spent years evaluating service-learning projects through my work with a wide range of undergraduate students, graduate students, and community partners, I can confidently say that service-learning offers powerful teaching and learning opportunities. As previously detailed, the time and effort that goes into planning for and executing service-learning projects is well worth it when you consider the incredible experiences and benefits experienced by everyone involved in the process, as reinforced by the emerging basis of evidence in this area. It is always exciting to see students realize the impacts of their own work in real-world contexts, and it is my hope that the foundation provided in this primer will facilitate the completion of many additional meaningful and rewarding service-learning projects in our fields!

Appendices

SAMPLE SERVICE-LEARNING FORMS

The sample forms and projects included in this section were originally developed based on personal experience and guidelines provided by the Office of Experiential Learning at the University of Central Florida to faculty members engaged in service-learning. These forms have been repeatedly modified and field tested over a period of approximately eight years. Although it is possible that some of these forms could be applicable to readers for immediate use, the intention in including the samples was to provide individual students and course instructors with "food for thought" as they develop their own tools that are relevant to individual course and project needs.

APPENDIX A:
SAMPLE SERVICE-LEARNING PROJECT DESCRIPTIONS
Undergraduate Augmentative and Alternative Communication Course

Project Option 1—Spring Fling Planning

Agency:	ABC Public Schools
Address:	123 Avenue A; City X
Activity:	Work with ABC staff members and speech–language pathologists to prepare for and publicize a full-day "Spring Fling" workshop on social skills for teenagers who use AAC and their parents on April 1.
Contact:	Amy Apple (Director)
Website:	http://www.xxx.xx
Phone:	xxx.xxx.xxxx
E-mail:	amyapple@xxx.com

Project Option 2—Assistive Technology Awareness Day Planning

Agency:	ABC Public Schools
Address:	123 Avenue A; City X
Activity:	Work with ABC staff members and speech–language pathologists to prepare for, publicize, and manage an Assistive Technology Awareness Day Exhibit at XYZ University on February 2.
Contact:	Amy Apple (Director)
Website:	http://www.xxx.xx
Phone:	xxx.xxx.xxxx
E-mail:	amyapple@xxx.com

Project Option 3—Software Presentation with ABC AT Staff

Agency: ABC Assistive Technology Network

Address: 1414 Street; City X

Activity: Work with DEF AT staff members to learn to use *Boardmaker©* and to plan and co-present a workshop for parents and teachers. It should be noted that prior software knowledge is not required; all necessary training will be provided.

Contact: Suzy Speech (Director)

Website: http://www.xxx.xx

Phone: xxx.xxx.xxxx

E-mail: Suzyspeech@xxx.com

Project Option 4—Classroom AAC Support

Agency: Sunny Skies Middle School

Address: 1234 Shiny Drive; City Y

Activity: Provide supplemental AAC services for students using AAC in a classroom context. Students will work with classroom teacher to identify convenient weekly or bi-weekly times to work in the classroom. Please note that a background check will be required.

Contact: Sandy Sunshine (Teacher)

Website: http://www.xxx.xx

Phone: xxx.xxx.xxxx

Fax: xxx.xxx.xxx

E-mail: SandySunshine@xxx.com

APPENDIX B:
SAMPLE SERVICE-LEARNING PROJECT CONTRACT

Contact Details
Student
Name: _____

Cell Phone: _____

Email: _____

Course Instructor
Name: _____

Office Phone: _____

Cell Phone: _____

Email: _____

Agency Contact/Site Supervisor
Name: _____

Location: _____

Office Phone: _____

Cell Phone: _____

Email: _____

Logistics
Expected Project Start Date: _____

Expected Project End Date: _____

Approximate Number of Hours per Week: _____

Other Details: _____

_____

_____

_____

_____

STUDENT AND AGENCY REPRESENTATIVE:

Service-Learning Assignment Description:

Provide a complete description of the service activities in which the student(s) will be engaged, including details of the products to be generated or services to be delivered by the student(s) and all agency expectations.

_____

_____

_____

_____

_____

_____

_____

Timeline

Project Milestone/Action/Deliverable	Deadline
Form a group and contract with instructor to select a service-learning project and agency.	*Date:* *(Latest Date = xx.xx.xx)*
Research information on agency and prepare for meeting with agency representative.	*Date:* *(Latest Date = xx.xx.xx)*
Meet with contact person from agency to develop service-learning assignment description (complete above).	*Date:* *(Latest Date = xx.xx.xx)*
Complete and submit *Service-Learning Assignment Contract* to course instructor.	*Date:* *(Latest Date = xx.xx.xx)*
Submit a detailed outline for how you plan to tackle the product or service that you will plan, develop, or deliver for your assigned community partner (e.g., set deadlines to submit product drafts to instructor and agency representative for feedback).	*Date:* *(Latest Date = xx.xx.xx)*

Project Milestone/Action/Deliverable	Deadline
Complete a reflection blog entry (as described in the syllabus) following each service-learning activity and group meeting.	*Date:* *(Latest Date = xx.xx.xx)*
Incorporate instructor and agency feedback when preparing the product or service plan and submit a first draft of product to the instructor along with the agency feedback you obtained on your outline to the course instructor.	*Date:* *(Latest Date = xx.xx.xx)*
Incorporate instructor feedback and submit a second draft of product or service plans to the agency.	*Date:* *(Latest Date = xx.xx.xx)*
Incorporate agency feedback and submit final product or other documentation of final product (e.g., video of presentation delivered, brochure developed, therapy summaries, etc.) to instructor and agency.	*Date:* *(Latest Date = xx.xx.xx)*
Give agency contact the assessment form and request that it be completed and returned by fax or e-mail to the course instructor by xx.xx.xx.	*Date:* *(Latest Date = xx.xx.xx)*
Submit individual Self/Peer Assessment Form to instructor.	*Date:* *(Latest Date = xx.xx.xx)*
Deliver 15-minute in-class presentation to summarize your service-learning project experiences. Include reflections on connections to course objectives.	*Date:* *(Latest Date = xx.xx.xx)*

* The instructor listed the latest possible deadlines for the completion/ submission of all project milestones above. Please note that each student must contract with his/her agency representative to determine firm deadlines for each milestone and enter the mutually agreed upon date above.

STUDENT:

I agree to abide by the following Guidelines and Limitations:

Guidelines

- **Ask for help when in doubt.** Your agency contact understands the issues at your site, and you are encouraged to approach him/her with problems or questions as they arise. He or she can assist you in determining the best way to respond to difficult or uncomfortable situations. You should also plan to contact your instructor when questions arise.
- **Be appropriate.** You are in a work situation and are expected to treat your supervisor and others with courtesy, respect, and kindness. Dress comfortably, neatly, and appropriately. Use formal names unless instructed otherwise. Set a positive standard for other students to follow to further the university's relationship with your agency.
- **Be flexible.** The level or intensity of activity at a service site is not always predictable. Your flexibility to changing situations can assist the partnership in working smoothly and producing positive outcomes for everyone involved.
- **Be punctual and responsible.** Although you are not a paid employee, you are participating in the organization as a reliable, trustworthy, and contributing member of the team. Both the administrators and the person with whom you will be working will rely on your punctuality and commitment to completing your service-learning project throughout your partnership.
- **Call if you anticipate lateness or absence.** Call the agency contact if you are unable to participate or if you anticipate being late.
- **Respect the privacy of all service providers.** If you are privy to confidential information with regard to the persons with whom you are working (e.g., organization files, cases, personal stories), it is vital that you treat everything as privileged information. You should use pseudonyms in your course assignments if you are referring to agency clients. You must abide by HIPAA requirements as relevant.
- **Show respect for your assigned community-based organization.** Placement within community programs is an educational opportunity and a privilege. Keep in mind that, in addition to your serving your community, your community is serving you by investing valuable resources in your learning.

Limitations

- **DO NOT:**
    - o Engage in any type of business with agency representatives or clients during the term of your service.
    - o Enter into personal relationships with clients or community partner representatives during the term of your service.
    - o Lend clients or coworkers money or other personal belongings, and do not borrow from clients or coworkers.
    - o Make promises or commitments you cannot keep.
    - o Report to your service site under the influence of drugs or alcohol.
    - o Tolerate or engage in interactions (verbal or otherwise) that might be perceived as sexual in nature.
    - o Tolerate or engage in interactions that might be perceived as discriminating against an individual or agency on any basis.
    - o Transport clients or agency representatives in personal vehicles.

*If you feel that your rights have been or may be violated, or that any of the above stated limitations have been violated, please contact the instructor and the following individual: _____.

I understand the connection between my academic course objectives and the service-learning assignment described above.

I have participated in any offered agency/class orientations and read the above stated guidelines and limitations and understand my role as a service-learning student in working with my assigned community partner.

I agree to act in a responsible manner while representing the university at the service-learning placement site and to abide by all rules and regulations that govern the site to which I have been assigned.

I understand and acknowledge the following risks involved with this service placement, and enter into this internship placement fully informed and aware.

Potential Risks:

1. _____

2. _____

3. _____

4. _____

I agree to devote at least _____ hours per week for an approximate total of _____ hours across the semester, in order to complete the above-described service-learning project/activities.

I agree to complete any forms, evaluations, or other paperwork required by either the course instructor or my assigned agency.

Student Signature: _____

Date: _____

<u>AGENCY CONTACT:</u>

I agree to guide this student's work, to provide ongoing feedback relative to the above project/activities and to submit a brief final evaluation of the student's achievement upon request.

I agree to discuss any concerns about the student's performance with him/her directly and with the course instructor if necessary.

Agency Contact Signature: _____

Date: _____

FACULTY MEMBER/COURSE INSTRUCTOR:

I have examined and approved this service-learning project contract/plan and will provide feedback and assistance throughout the duration of this project.

Course Instructor Signature: _____

Date: _____

APPENDIX C:
SAMPLE SERVICE-LEARNING ACTIVITY HOUR LOG

Date	Description of Service-Learning Activities	Time Spent
Total Number of Hours		

Student Name and Group: _____

Student Signature: _____

Agency Contact Name: _____

Agency Contact Signature: _____

Date: _____

APPENDIX D:
WEEKLY REFLECTION TOOL

Student Name: _____

Reflection Week: _____

Description of Service-Learning Activities during the Week *(What happened?)*	**Feelings and Reactions** *(How did you feel?)*
Connections to Course Objectives *(How did your SL activities this week connect to the course content?)*	**Next Steps** *(What actions will you take next?)*

APPENDIX E:
SAMPLE SERVICE-LEARNING AGENCY EVALUATION FORM

Agency Name: _____

Contact Person: _____

E-mail: _____ Phone: _____

Please indicate your level of agreement with the below statements.

1	2	3	4	5
Disagree	**Somewhat Disagree**	**Neutral**	**Agree**	**Strongly Agree**

	1	2	3	4	5
A. The students who worked with my agency respected the opinions of agency staff and/or clients and incorporated agency suggestions/feedback/requests.	1	2	3	4	5
B. The students who worked with my agency conducted themselves in a professional manner and took their work seriously (e.g., communication, conduct, dress, punctuality).	1	2	3	4	5
C. The students who worked with my agency were committed to excellence in their work.	1	2	3	4	5
D. The students who worked with my agency demonstrated the expected knowledge and skills relevant to the project.	1	2	3	4	5
E. I developed or confirmed a positive impression of university students through this project.	1	2	3	4	5

1	2	3	4	5
Disagree	Somewhat Disagree	Neutral	Agree	Strongly Agree

F. The benefits my agency received from this project made it worth my time commitment.	1	2	3	4	5
G. I would participate in a service-learning project with university students again and recommend a similar experience to others.	1	2	3	4	5
H. My experience with service-learning this semester was worthwhile.	1	2	3	4	5
Total Points	__ /40				

Please provide written comments to explain the above ratings and any suggestions you may have for future projects on a separate piece of paper.

APPENDIX F:
SAMPLE SERVICE-LEARNING SELF/PEER EVALUATION FORM

Student Name: _____

Group Assignment: _____

Self- and Peer-Rating Categories

    A. Communication Skills
    B. Punctuality and Availability for Meetings
    C. Dependability to Get Tasks Accomplished
    D. Ability to Collaborate with Team Members
    E. Ability to Work with People Outside Group (e.g., instructor, agency contact)
    F. Leadership Skills
    G. Demonstrated Ability at Generating Ideas
    H. Demonstrated Ability at Developing Others' Ideas
    I. Demonstrated Ability at Incorporating Feedback
    J. Demonstrated Ability at Generating Written Materials

1. Considering the above categories and any others you identify as relevant, describe your own and your peer(s)' major contributions to the service-learning project.

Your Major Contribution	Peer 1 (Name):	Peer 2 (Name):

2. Considering the categories on page 1 (of this form) and any others you identify as relevant, describe your own and your peer(s)' greatest strengths as service-learning team members for this project.

Your Greatest Strength	Peer 1 (Name):	Peer 2 (Name):

3. Considering the categories on page 1 and any others you identify as relevant, what do you think you or your peer(s) could have done better while working on this project?

What You Could Have Improved	Peer 1 (Name):	Peer 2 (Name):

4. Please add any additional comments about your work or the work of your peer(s) for this service learning project.

Your Work	Peer 1 (Name):	Peer 2 (Name):

5. What Grade would you give yourself and your peer(s) on this project and why? (A, A–, B+, B, B–, C+, C, D, F)

Your Grade	Peer 1 (Name):	Peer 2 (Name):

REFERENCES

American Speech-Language-Hearing Association. (2005). *Roles and responsibilities of speech-language pathologists with respect to augmentative and alternative communication: Position statement.* Available from www.asha.org/policy

American Speech-Language-Hearing Assocation. (2011a). *ASHA federal advocacy issues.* Retrieved from www.asha.org/advocacy/briefs-agenda

American Speech-Language-Hearing Association. (2011b). *Career information.* Retrieved from www.asha.org/careers/professions/default-overview.htm

Astin, A. W., & Sax, L. J. (1998). How undergraduates are affected by service participation. *Journal of College Student Development, 39*(3), 251–263.

Bailey, R. L., & Angell, M. E. (2005). Service learning in speech–language pathology: Stakeholders' perceptions of a school-based feeding improvement project. *Contemporary Issues in Communication Science and Disorders, 32,* 126–133.

Balazadeh, N. (1996). *Service-learning and the sociological imagination: Approach and assessment.* Paper presented at the National Historically Black Colleges and Universities Faculty Development Symposium, Memphis, TN.

Batchelder, T. H., & Root, S. (1994). Effects of an undergraduate program to integrate academic learning and service: Cognitive, prosocial cognitive, and identity outcomes. *Journal of Adolescence, 17,* 341–355.

Berger Kaye, C. (2004). *The complete guide to service learning: Proven, practical ways to engage students in civic responsibility, academic curriculum, & social action.* Minneapolis, MN: Free Spirit Publishing.

Binger, C., & Kent-Walsh, J. (2010). *What every speech–language pathologist/audiologist should know about augmentative and alternative communication.* Boston: Pearson Education.

Bowdon, M. (2005, March). *When the radical becomes familiar: The pros and cons of institutionalizing service-learning.* Conference on College Composition and Communication. San Francisco, CA.

Boyatzis, R. E. (1998). *Transforming Qualitative Information.* Thousand Oaks, CA: Sage Publications.

Campus Compact. (2007). *2006 Service statistics: Highlights and trends from Campus Compact's Annual Membership Survey.* Boston: Author.

Dictionary.com. (2011a). Retrieved from http://dictionary.reference.com/browse/learning

Dictionary.com. (2011b). Retrieved from http://dictionary.reference.com/browse/service

Eyler, J., & Giles, D. E. (1994). The theoretical roots of service-learning in John Dewey: Toward a theory of service-learning. *Michigan Journal of Community Service Learning, 1*(1), 77–78.

Eyler, J., & Giles, D. E. (1999). *Where's the learning in service-learning?* San Francisco, CA: Jossey-Bass Publishers.

Eyler, J. S., Giles, D. E., Stenson, C. M., & Gray, C. J. (2001). *At a glance: What we know about the effects of service-learning on college students, faculty, institutions and communities, 1993–2000: Third edition.* Retrieved from www.compact.org/wp-content/uploads/resources/downloads/aag.pdf

Goldberg, L. R., Richburg, C. M., & Wood, L. A. (2006). Active learning through service-learning. *Communication Disorders Quarterly, 27*(3), 131–145.

Hurd, C. (2007). *Colorado State University Service-Learning Faculty Manual, Fourth Edition.* Retrieved from http://tilt.colostate.edu/guides/tilt_servicelearning

Kendrick, R. J. (1996). Outcomes of service-learning in an introduction to sociology course. *Michigan Journal of Community Service Learning, 3,* 72–81.

Kent-Walsh, J. (2005, November). *TeenTech: A service-learning approach to undergraduate instruction in AAC.* Poster presented at the Annual Convention of the American Speech-Language-Hearing Association, San Diego, CA.

Mabry, J. B. (1998). Pedagogical variations in service-learning and student outcomes: How time, contact, and reflection matter. *Michigan Journal of Community Service Learning, 5,* 32–47.

Mintz, S., & Hesser, G. (1996). Principles of good practice in service learning. In B. Jacoby & Associates (Eds.), *Service-learning in higher education* (pp. 26–51). San Francisco, CA: Jossey-Bass Publishers.

Myers-Lipton, S. J. (1996). Effect of service-learning on college students' attitudes toward international understanding. *Journal of College Student Development, 37*(6), 659–668.

National Service-Learning Clearinghouse. (2011a). *Higher education community engagement quality practices.* Retrieved from www.servicelearning.org/topic/quality-components-standards /he-community-engagement-quality-practices

National Service-Learning Clearinghouse. (2011b). *What is service-learning?* Retrieved from http://www.servicelearning.org/what-is-service-learning

Scherz, J. (2008). A service learning project in AAC. *Perspectives on Augmentative and Alternative Communication, 17,* 140–143.

Seifer, S. D., and Connors, K., Eds. (2007). Community Campus Partnerships for Health. *Faculty toolkit for service-learning in higher education.* Scotts Valley, CA: National Service-Learning Clearinghouse.

Steinberg, K. S., Bringle, R. G., & Williams, M. J. (2010). *Service-learning research primer.* Scotts Valley, CA: National Service-Learning Clearinghouse.

University of Central Florida. (2007). *Criteria and procedures for service learning course approval.* Retrieved from www.explearning.ucf.edu/UserFiles/File/SL%20course%20approval%20criteria%20procedure%20as%20of%202007.doc

University of Central Florida. (2011). *Service-Learning Overview.* Retrieved from http://www.explearning.ucf.edu/categories/For%20Faculty/Service-Learning/147_146.aspx

University of Minnesota. (2011). *Types of community engagement.* Retrieved from www.morris.umn.edu/communityengagement/types/

Vogelgesang, L. J., & Astin, A. W. (2000). Comparing the effects of community service and service-learning. *Michigan Journal of Community Service Learning, 7,* 25–34.